EATING HEALTHY WITH DR. FRANCIS

---

28 DAY

VEGETARIAN
Weight Loss Plan

Dr. A. Francis

December | 2022

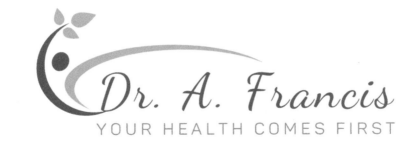

CONTENTS

MEAL PLANS

- Essential Ingredients 5
- WEEK 1 Meal Plan 6
- WEEK 1 Grocery List 7
- WEEK 2 Meal Plan 8
- WEEK 2 Grocery List 9
- WEEK 3 Meal Plan 10
- WEEK 3 Grocery List 11
- WEEK 4 Meal Plan 12
- WEEK 4 Grocery List 13

CONTENTS

RECIPES

- Green Smoothie 14
- Raspberry Smoothie 15
- Chocolate Smoothie 16
- Blueberry Smoothie 17
- Superfood Oatmeal 18
- Overnight Oats 19
- Mexican Scramble 20
- Apple Cereal 21
- Banana Pancakes 22
- Chickpea Wrap 23
- Arugula Salad 24
- Broccoli Soup 25
- Falafel Salad 26
- Greek Salad 27
- Kale Salad 28
- Quinoa Tabbouleh 29
- Stuffed Avocados 30
- Buddha Bowl 31
- Tomato Pasta 32
- Bean Burger 33
- Chickpea Curry 34
- Stuffed Sweet Potato 35
- Lentil Meatballs 36
- Kelp Noodle Stir Fry 37
- Tofu Pad Thai 38
- Chickpea Burger 39
- Vegetarian Fajitas 40
- Tuscan Bean Stew 41
- Broccoli Quinoa Cakes 42
- Hummus Cucumbers 43
- Carrots & Nut Butter 44
- Crackers & Guacamole 45
- Cacao Coconut Balls 46
- Apple Pie Bites 47
- Superfood Cookies 48
- Easy Trail Mix 49
- Berry Chia Pudding 50

ESSENTIAL INGREDIENTS

CONDIMENTS

- Marinara Sauce
- Tahini
- Sundried Tomatoes
- Olive Oil
- Breadcrumbs
- Tomato purée
- Onion powder
- Paprika
- Ground Cumin
- Balsamic Vinegar
- Coconut Aminos
- Almond Butter
- Vegan Mayo
- Italian Herbs
- Mix Seasoning
- Chilli Powder
- Cayenne Powder
- Coconut Oil
- Ground Turmeric
- Ground Ginger

PROTEIN POWDER

- Vanilla Protein Powder
- Chocolate Protein Powder

NUTS & SEEDS

- Almonds
- Pumpkin Seeds
- Walnuts
- Ground Flax Seeds
- Chia Seeds
- Pine Nuts
- Cashews
- Sesame Seeds
- Sunflower Seeds

BAKING SUPPLIES

- Almond Flour
- Coconut Chips
- Maple Syrup
- Apple Chips
- Medjool Dates
- Cinnamon
- Dried Cranberries
- Baking Powder
- Vanilla Extract
- Raw Cacao Powder
- Raisins
- Shredded Coconut

MEAL PLAN WEEK 1

Use extra serving from previous day.

	MONDAY	TUESDAY	WEDNESDAY	THURSDAY	FRIDAY	SATURDAY	SUNDAY
BREAKFAST	Green Protein Smoothie page 14	Superfood Oatmeal page 18	Raspberry Coconut Smoothie page 15	Superfood Oatmeal page 18	Green Protein Smoothie page 14	Superfood Oatmeal page 18	Banana Pancakes page 22
LUNCH	Chickpea Wrap page 23	Buddha Bowl * page 31	Balsamic Arugula Salad * page 24	Creamy Tomato Pasta * page 32	Tofu Pad Thai * page 38	Caprese Stuffed Avocados page 30	Chickpea Curry * page 34
SNACK	Hummus Cucumber Sticks page 43	Cacao Coconut Balls page 46	Hummus Cucumber Sticks page 43	Cacao Coconut Balls page 46	Hummus Cucumber Sticks page 43	Cacao Coconut Balls page 46	Hummus Cucumber Sticks page 43
DINNER	Buddha Bowl page 31	Balsamic Arugula Salad page 24	Creamy Tomato Pasta page 32	Tofu Pad Thai page 38	Vegetarian Fajitas page 40	Chickpea Curry page 34	Kelp Noodle Stir Fry page 37

GROCERY LIST

VEGETABLES

- 5 Avocados
- 1 Lemon
- 6 Cups Spinach
- 4 Cups Arugula
- 1 Small Sweet Potato
- 1 Head Broccoli
- 2 Carrots
- 2 ½ Red Bell Peppers
- 1 Stalk Celery
- 2 English Cucumbers
- 2 Tomatoes
- ¼ Cup Cherry Tomatoes
- 1 Cup Bean Sprouts
- ½ Cup Green Onions
- 4 Onions
- 5 Clove Garlic
- ½ Cup Mushrooms

FRUITS & BERRIES

- 5 Bananas
- ½ Cup Mixed Berries
- 1 Cup Raspberries

GRAINS, LEGUMES, CANS

- ¼ Cup Black Beans
- 5 ½ Cup Gluten-Free Oats
- 2 Brown Rice Tortillas
- 7 oz Brown Rice Pasta
- 2 Cups Cooked Quinoa
- 4 Cans Chickpeas
- 2 Cans Diced Tomatoes

DAIRY, MILK, SOY PRODUCTS

- ¼ Cup Mini Mozzarella Balls
- 10 oz Tempeh
- 7 oz Kelp Noodles
- 1 Cup Coconut Milk
- 5 ¾ Cups Almond Milk
- 10 oz Tofu

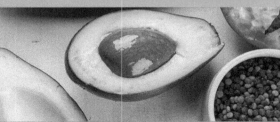

MEAL PLAN WEEK 2

Use extra serving from previous day.

	MONDAY	TUESDAY	WEDNESDAY	THURSDAY	FRIDAY	SATURDAY	SUNDAY
BREAKFAST	Raspberry Coconut Smoothie *page 15*	Carrot Overnight Oats *page 19*	Green Protein Smoothie *page 14*	Carrot Overnight Oats *page 19*	Raspberry Coconut Smoothie *page 15*	Carrot Overnight Oats *page 19*	Banana Pancake *page 22*
LUNCH	Kelp Noodle Stir Fry * *page 37*	Creamy Broccoli Soup * *page 25*	Falafel Salad * *page 26*	Stuffed Sweet Potato * *page 35*	Black Bean Burgers * *page 33*	Crunchy Kale Salad *page 28*	Zoodles & Lentil Meatballs *page 36*
SNACK	Seed Crackers & Guacamole *page 45*	Carrots & Almond Butter *page 44*	Seed Crackers & Guacamole *page 45*	Carrots & Almond Butter *page 44*	Seed Crackers & Guacamole *page 45*	Carrots & Almond Butter *page 44*	Seed Crackers Guacamo *page 45*
DINNER	Creamy Broccoli Soup *page 25*	Falafel Salad *page 26*	Stuffed Sweet Potato *page 35*	Black Bean Burgers *page 33*	Chickpea Burger *page 39*	Zoodles & Lentil Meatballs *page 36*	Quinoa Tabboule *page 29*

GROCERY LIST WEEK 2

VEGETABLES

- 1 Lemon
- 2 Limes
- 2 Cups Kale
- 2 Cup Fresh Greens
- 1 ¼ Cup Fresh Parsley
- ½ Cup Cilantro
- 2 Sweet Potatoes
- ½ Avocado
- 1 Head of Broccoli
- 8 Carrots
- 2 Zucchinis
- 4 Tomatoes
- 2 Leeks
- 2 Onions
- 7 Cloves Garlic
- ½ Cucumber
- ½ Cup Lettuce
- 1 Cup Spinach

FRUITS & BERRIES

- 2 Cups Raspberries
- 3 Bananas

GRAINS, LEGUMES, CANS

- 2 Cans Chickpeas
- 2 ¾ Cup Gluten-Free Oats
- ½ Cup Quinoa
- 1 Can Black Beans
- 1 Cup Corn
- 1 Cup Cooked Lentils
- 4 Cups Vegetable Broth

DAIRY, MILK, EGGS

- 3 Cups Coconut Milk
- 2 ½ Cups Almond Milk
- 1 egg

MEAL PLAN WEEK 3

Use extra serving from previous day.

	MONDAY	TUESDAY	WEDNESDAY	THURSDAY	FRIDAY	SATURDAY	SUNDAY
BREAKFAST	Chocolate Banana Smoothie *page 16*	Mexican Scramble *page 20*	Blueberry Smoothie *page 17*	Mexican Scramble *page 20*	Chocolate Banana Smoothie *page 16*	Mexican Scramble *page 20*	Banana Pancakes *page 22*
LUNCH	Quinoa * Tabbouleh *page 29*	Buddha Bowl * *page 31*	Balsamic Arugula Salad * *page 24*	Creamy Tomato Pasta * *page 32*	Tofu Pad Thai * *page 38*	Caprese Stuffed Avocados *page 30*	Chickpea Curry * *page 34*
SNACK	Coconut Chia Pudding *page 50*	Apple Pie Bites *page 47*	Coconut Chia Pudding *page 50*	Apple Pie Bites *page 47*	Coconut Chia Pudding *page 50*	Apple Pie Bites *page 47*	Coconut Chia Pudding *page 50*
DINNER	Buddha Bowl *page 31*	Balsamic Arugula Salad *page 24*	Creamy Tomato Pasta *page 32*	Tofu Pad Thai *page 38*	Broccoli Quinoa Cakes *page 42*	Chickpea Curry *page 34*	Kelp Noodle Stir Fry *page 37*

GROCERY LIST WEEK 3

VEGETABLES

- 1 Lemon
- 4 Cups Spinach
- 4 Cups Arugula
- 2 Small Sweet Potatoes
- 2 Carrots
- 4 Red Bell Pepper
- ¼ Cup Red Cabbage
- ½ Cup Green Onions
- 2 Tomatoes
- ¼ Cup Cherry Tomatoes
- 1 Stalk Celery
- 1 Cup Bean Sprouts
- 4 ½ Avocados
- 3 Onions
- 5 Garlic Cloves
- ¼ Cup Fresh Herbs
- ¼ Cup Lettuce
- 2 Broccoli Heads
- 1 Cucumber

FRUITS & BERRIES

- 6 Bananas
- 1 Cup Mixed Berries
- 1 Cup Blueberries

GRAINS, LEGUMES, CANS

- 3 Cups Gluten-Free Oats
- 7 oz Kelp Noodles
- 1 Brown Rice Tortillas
- 7 oz Brown Rice Pasta
- 2 ½ Cups Cooked Quinoa
- 3 Cans Chickpeas
- 1 Can Black Beans
- 2 Cans Diced Tomatoes

DAIRY, MILK, SOY PRODUCTS

- 1 tbsp Grated Cheese
- 7 eggs
- 2 Cans Coconut Milk
- 10 oz Tempeh
- 10 oz Tofu
- 2 ¾ Cups Almond Milk
- ¼ Cup Mozzarella

MEAL PLAN WEEK 4

Use extra serving from previous day.

	MONDAY	TUESDAY	WEDNESDAY	THURSDAY	FRIDAY	SATURDAY	SUNDAY
BREAKFAST	Blueberry Smoothie *page 17*	Apple Cinnamon Cereal *page 21*	Chocolate Banana Smoothie *page 16*	Apple Cinnamon Cereal *page 21*	Blueberry Smoothie *page 17*	Apple Cinnamon Cereal *page 21*	Banana Pancake *page 22*
LUNCH	Kelp Noodle Stir Fry * *page 37*	Creamy Broccoli Soup * *page 25*	Falafel Salad * *page 26*	Stuffed Sweet Potato * *page 35*	Black Bean Burgers * *page 33*	Crunchy Kale Salad *page 28*	Zoodles & Lentil Meatballs *page 36*
SNACK	Seed Crackers & Guacamole *page 45*	Carrots & Almond Butter *page 44*	Seed Crackers & Guacamole *page 45*	Carrots & Almond Butter *page 44*	Seed Crackers & Guacamole *page 45*	Carrots & Almond Butter *page 44*	Seed Crackers & Guacamole *page 45*
DINNER	Creamy Broccoli Soup *page 25*	Falafel Salad *page 26*	Stuffed Sweet Potato *page 35*	Black Bean Burgers *page 33*	Tuscan Bean Stew *page 41*	Zoodles & Lentil Meatballs *page 36*	Quinoa Tabbouleh *page 29*

GROCERY LIST WEEK 4

VEGETABLES

- 2½ Avocados
- 1 Lemon
- 2 Tbsp Lime Juice
- 2 ½ Cups Kale
- 2 Cup Fresh Greens
- 1 ¼ Cup Fresh Parsley
- 2 Small Sweet Potatoes
- 1 Head of Broccoli
- 2 Carrots
- 2 Zucchinis
- 4 Tomatoes
- 2½ Leeks
- 1 Red Onion
- 2 Onions
- 8 Cloves Garlic
- ½ Cup Cilantro
- ½ Stick Celery

FRUITS & BERRIES

- 5 Bananas
- 3 Apples
- 2 Cups Blueberries

GRAINS, LEGUMES, CANS

- 2 ¾ Cup Gluten-Free Oats
- 1/2 Cup Quinoa
- 2 Cans Black Beans
- 2 Cans Chickpeas
- 1 Cup Cooked Lentils
- 1 Cup Corn
- 3 Cups Vegetable Broth
- 5 oz Borlotti Beans

DAIRY, MILK, SOY PRODUCTS

- 1 Can Coconut Milk
- 2 ¾ Cups Almond Milk

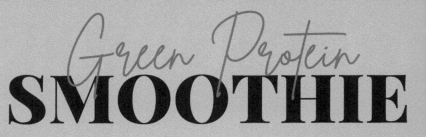

Green Protein SMOOTHIE

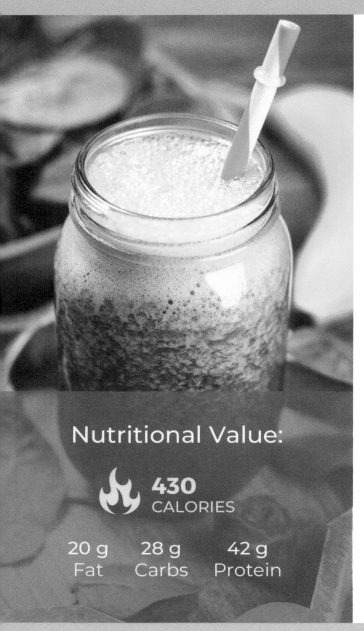

Nutritional Value:

430 CALORIES

20 g Fat   28 g Carbs   42 g Protein

INGREDIENTS

- ½ frozen banana
- 1 cup spinach
- ½ avocado
- 1 scoop vanilla protein powder
- 1 cup almond milk
- 1 tbsp chia seeds

DIRECTIONS

1. Pour the almond milk into the blender.

2. Add in the banana, avocado, spinach, chia seeds, protein powder.

3. Turn the blender on, starting at a low speed, and increase as needed.

4. Once the liquid looks smooth, pour into a cup and enjoy immediately.

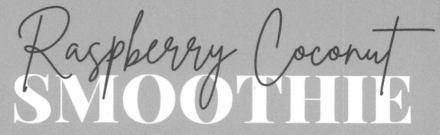

Raspberry Coconut
SMOOTHIE

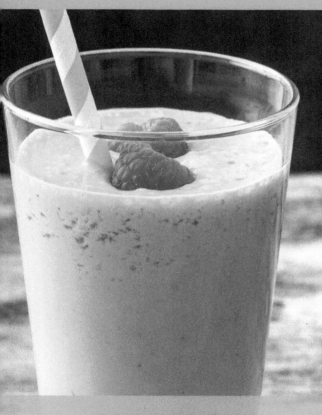

Nutritional Value:

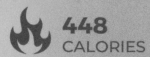 **448** CALORIES

10 g Fat **54 g** Carbs **41 g** Protein

INGREDIENTS

- 1 cup raspberries
- ½ frozen banana
- 1 tbsp chia seeds
- 1 cup coconut milk
- 1 scoop vanilla protein powder

DIRECTIONS

1. Pour the coconut milk into the blender.

2. Add in the banana, raspberries, chia seeds, and protein powder

3. Turn the blender on, starting at a low speed, and increase as needed.

4. Once the liquid looks smooth, pour into a cup and enjoy immediately.

Chocolate Banana
SMOOTHIE

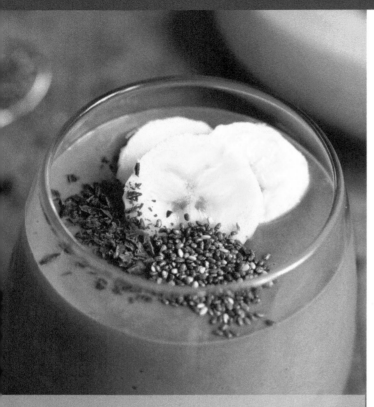

Nutritional Value:

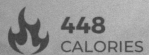 **448** CALORIES

10 g Fat

54 g Carbs

41 g Protein

INGREDIENTS

- 1 frozen banana
- ½ avocado
- 1 cup almond milk
- 1 tbsp cocoa powder
- 1 scoop chocolate protein powder

DIRECTIONS

1. Pour the almond milk into the blender.

2. Add in banana, avocado, cocoa powder, and protein powder.

3. Turn the blender on, starting at a low speed, and increase as needed.

4. Once the liquid looks smooth, pour into a cup and enjoy immediately.

Blueberry SMOOTHIE

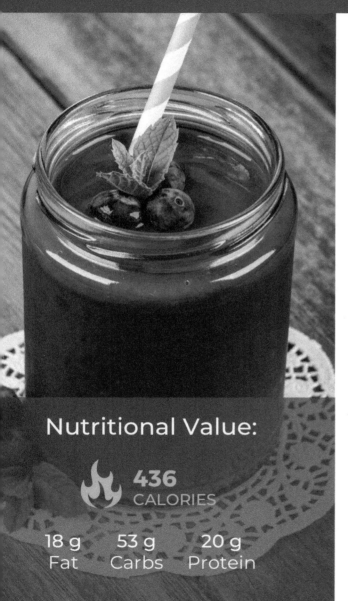

Nutritional Value:

436 CALORIES

| 18 g | 53 g | 20 g |
| Fat | Carbs | Protein |

INGREDIENTS

- 1 cup blueberries
- 1 banana
- 1 cup coconut milk
- 1 scoop vanilla protein powder
- Handful ice

DIRECTIONS

1. Pour the coconut milk into the blender.

2. Add in the blueberries, protein powder, banana and ice.

3. Turn the blender on, starting at a low speed, and increase as needed.

4. Once the liquid looks smooth, pour into a cup and enjoy immediately.

2 min
Prep

 20 min
Cook

1
Serving

Superfood
OATMEAL

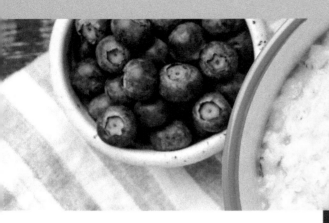 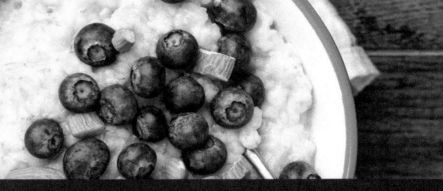

INGREDIENTS

- ½ cup gluten-free oats
- 1 cup almond milk
- 2 tbsp almonds
- ½ cup berries
- 1 tsp cinnamon

Nutritional Value:

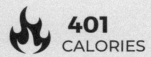 **401**
CALORIES

21 g
Fat

40 g
Carbs

12 g
Protein

DIRECTIONS

1. In a pot place the oats, cinnamon, and almond milk and turn the heat on high until it starts boiling.

2. Once it is boiling turn the heat down to low and stir until all the almond milk is absorbed.

3. Once the oatmeal is ready transfer it into a bowl and add the nuts and fresh berries. Optional: Add honey or extra toppings.

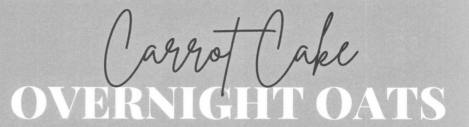

Carrot Cake
OVERNIGHT OATS

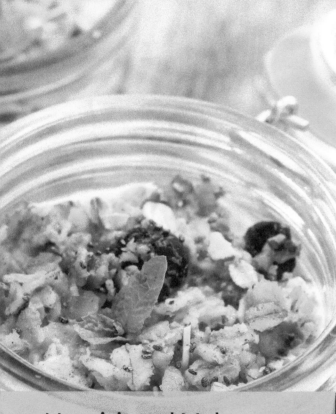

INGREDIENTS

- ½ cup gluten-free oats
- ¾ cup almond milk
- ¼ cup carrots, shredded
- ¼ cup walnuts
- 2 tbsp raisins
- 1 tbsp maple syrup
- ½ tsp cinnamon
- ⅛ tsp ginger

DIRECTIONS

1. Combine all the ingredients into a mason jar or a sealed container, give it a good stir, and place it in the fridge overnight.

2. In the morning, add an extra tablespoon of walnuts for an extra crunch if desired. Enjoy cold or warmed-up.

Nutritional Value:

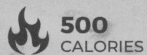

500 CALORIES

25 g Fat

78 g Carbs

11 g Protein

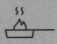

10 min
Prep

15 min
Cook

1
Serving

Mexican
SCRAMBLE

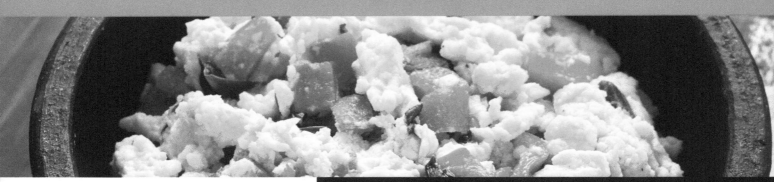

INGREDIENTS

- 2 eggs
- ½ cup sweet potatoes
- ½ cup black beans
- ½ cup red peppers
- 1 tsp coconut oil
- ½ avocado

Nutritional Value:

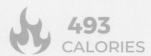 **493**
CALORIES

26 g
Fat

44 g
Carbs

23 g
Protein

DIRECTIONS

1. Heat a pan on medium heat and add the coconut oil.

2. Once the coconut oil is melted, add in the diced sweet potatoes and red pepper. Cover and cook for 8 minutes.

3. Once the sweet potatoes are soft, add in the black beans for 2 minutes to heat up. Add the 2 eggs, salt to taste and stir into a scramble.

4. Once the scramble is done, top it with avocado and hot sauce.

2 min Prep

 20 min Cook

 1 Serving

Apple Cinnamon CEREAL

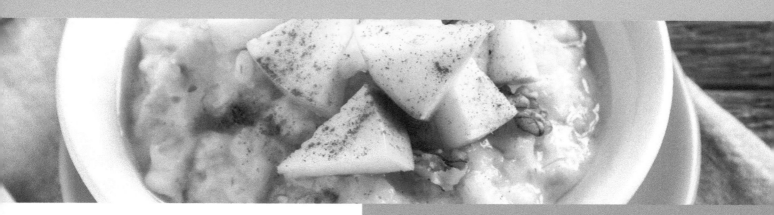

INGREDIENTS

- 1 apple
- ¼ cup coconut chips
- ½ cup almond milk
- 2 tbsp walnuts
- 2 tbsp almonds
- ½ tsp cinnamon

Nutritional Value:

 **350** CALORIES

28 g Fat

19 g Carbs

8 g Protein

DIRECTIONS

1. Start by washing an apple and then cut it into small pieces.

2. Next, combine the apple pieces and all the remaining ingredients into a small bowl.

3. Add any other nuts and seeds that you enjoy to add texture to this grain-free cereal.

2 min
Prep

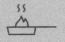 **10 min**
Cook

 1
Serving

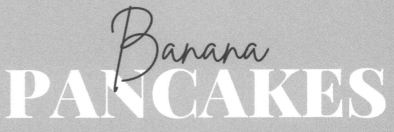

Banana
PANCAKES

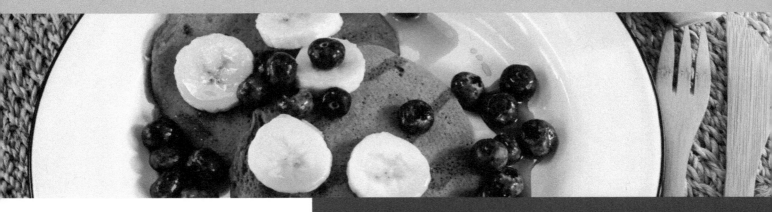

INGREDIENTS

- 1 banana
- 2 eggs
- 1 tsp cinnamon
- 1 tsp coconut oil

Nutritional Value:

 **378**
CALORIES

24 g
Fat

30 g
Carbs

14 g
Protein

DIRECTIONS

1. In a bowl combine the banana and two eggs. Use a hand blender or a fork to mix the banana and eggs.

2. Place a pan on medium heat and melt the coconut oil. Slowly add the batter to the pan forming 5-inch diameter pancakes. Place the cover on and cook for a couple of minutes on each side.

3. Repeat until you have cooked the whole batch. Be creative with your toppings, add any of your favorite clean foods.

2 min
Prep

 2 min
Cook

 1
Servings

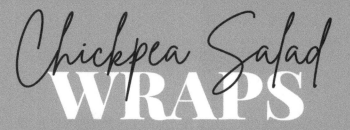
Chickpea Salad
WRAPS

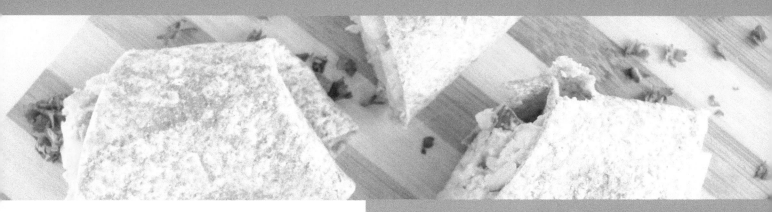

INGREDIENTS

- 1 brown rice tortilla
- ½ (15oz) can chickpeas
- ¼ avocado
- ½ stalk celery
- ¼ cup onions
- 2 tbsp vegan mayo

Nutritional Value:

 **359**
CALORIES

9 g
Fat

39.3 g
Carbs

9 g
Protein

DIRECTIONS

1. Wash and drain the chickpeas. Put the chickpeas in a big bowl & mash them with a fork.

2. Chop the celery and red onion into small pieces, then add them to the chickpeas.

3. Toss in the remaining ingredients. Top tortilla with mixture and roll up.

2 min
Prep

35 min
Cook

2
Servings *

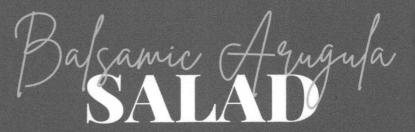

Balsamic Arugula
SALAD

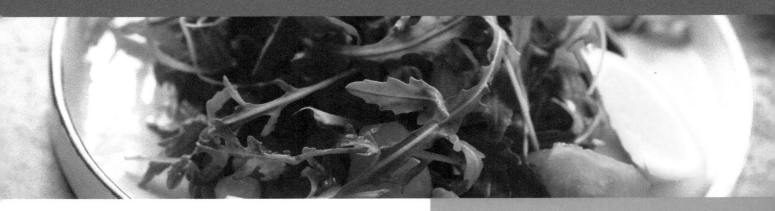

INGREDIENTS

- 4 cups arugula
- 2 tomatoes
- 1 cup cucumber
- 1 cup chickpeas
- 2 tbsp balsamic vinegar
- ¼ cup olive oil

Nutritional Value:

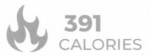 **391**
CALORIES

29 g
Fat

28 g
Carbs

6 g
Protein

DIRECTIONS

1. Preheat the oven to 400°F. Spread drained chickpeas on a baking sheet and drizzle 2 tbsp of olive oil on top. Bake for 30 minutes.

2. Make the dressing by combining the balsamic vinegar, olive oil, salt to taste

3. Once the chickpeas are done toss them into the prepared salad.

* *Refrigerate one serving.*

5 min
Prep

25 min
Cook

2 Servings *

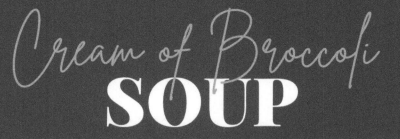

Cream of Broccoli
SOUP

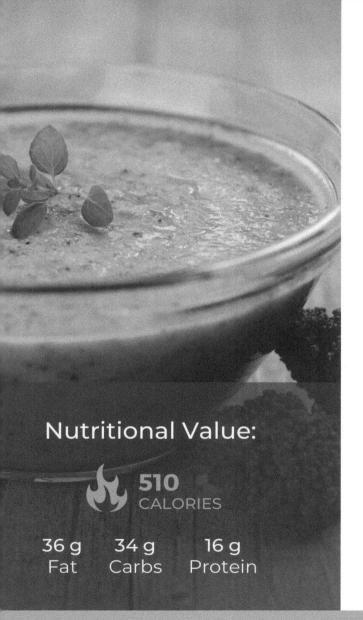

Nutritional Value:

510
CALORIES

36 g
Fat

34 g
Carbs

16 g
Protein

INGREDIENTS

- 1 head broccoli
- 2 leeks
- 4 cups vegetable broth
- 1 cup coconut milk
- ½ cup yellow onions
- 2 garlic cloves
- 1 tbsp olive oil

DIRECTIONS

1. Heat the olive oil in a pot on medium heat. Add in the onions and sauté for a few minutes. Add the garlic, sauté for 2 minutes. Next add the broccoli, salt to taste, leeks, and vegetable broth. Bring everything to a boil, then lower to a simmer for 20 minutes.

2. Add in the coconut milk, let it warm-up. Blend until smooth.

*** Refrigerate one serving.**

5 min
Prep

45 min
Cook

2
Servings *

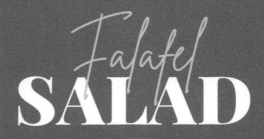

Falafel SALAD

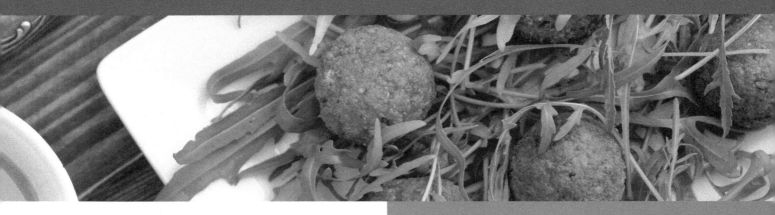

INGREDIENTS

- 1 can (15oz) chickpeas
- ½ cup onion
- 1 cup parsley
- 2 tbsp flax seed
- ½ tsp cumin
- 2 cups spring mix
- 1 tbsp tahini

Nutritional Value:

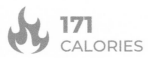 **171** CALORIES

3 g Fat   **29 g** Carbs   **9 g** Protein

DIRECTIONS

1. Combine the chickpeas, onions, flax seed, parsley, cumin, salt to taste in a food processor. Proces for a few seconds, leaving the mixture a little bit chunky.

2. Preheat the oven to 400°F. Form 8 small patties with the mixture. Bake for 45 minutes, flipping them halfway.

3. Prepare the salad by combining the tahini and spring mix.

* *Refrigerate one serving.*

5 min
Prep

5 min
Cook

2
Servings *

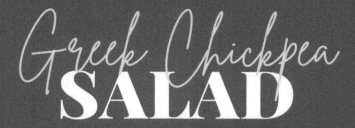

Greek Chickpea
SALAD

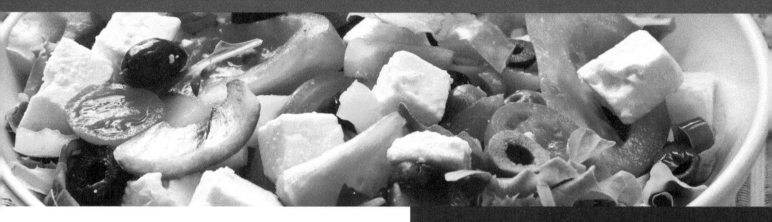

INGREDIENTS

- 2 cups chickpeas
- 2 tomatoes
- 1 cup cucumbers
- 2 tsp olive oil
- ½ cup feta cheese
- ¼ cup onions
- 12 olives

Nutritional Value:

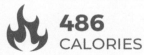 **486**
CALORIES

28 g
Fat

45 g
Carbs

16 g
Protein

DIRECTIONS

1. Prepare the vegetables by washing and slicing them. Drain and rinse the chickpeas.

2. Combine all the ingredients in a bowl. Drizzle the olive oil on top and add a pinch of salt and pepper to taste.

*** Refrigerate one serving.**

5 min Prep   **35 min** Cook   **2 Servings** *

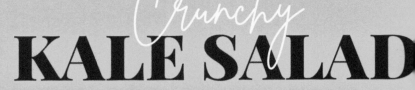
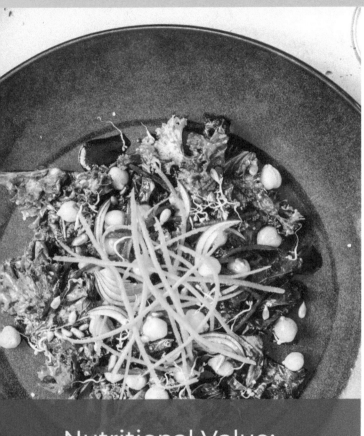

INGREDIENTS

- 4 cups kale
- 1 carrot
- 1 avocado
- 1 cup chickpeas
- 2 tbsp tahini
- 1 tbsp lemon juice

DIRECTIONS

1. Preheat the oven to 400°F. Spread drained chickpeas on a baking sheet. Bake for 30 minutes.

2. Meanwhile prepare vegetables by chopping up the kale, shredding the carrot, cutting the avocado into small cubes.

3. Place all the vegetables in a bowl with the baked chickpeas and then drizzle tahini and lemon juice

* Refrigerate one serving.

Nutritional Value:

 431 CALORIES

22 g Fat   **40 g** Carbs   **16 g** Protein

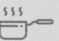

5 min
Prep

25 min
Cook

2
Servings *

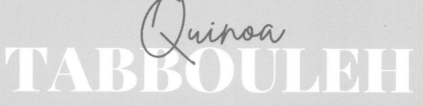

Quinoa TABBOULEH

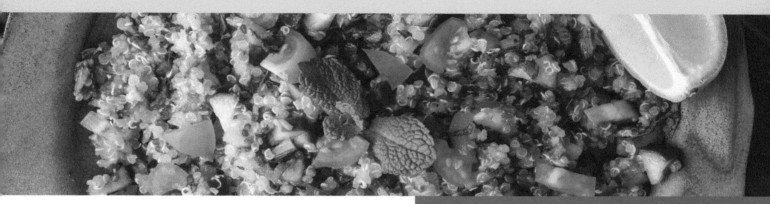

INGREDIENTS

- ½ cup quinoa
- 1 cup fresh parsley
- 4 tomatoes
- 4 tbsp pine nuts
- 2 tbsp tahini
- 2 tbsp olive oil
- Juice of 1 lemon

DIRECTIONS

1. Start by preparing the quinoa according to the directions on the packaging.

2. While the quinoa is cooking start chopping the parsley and the tomatoes.

3. Once the quinoa is done let it cool down for a little bit and then add all the remaining ingredients. Mix well and serve cold.

* *Refrigerate one serving.*

Nutritional Value:

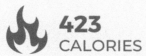 **423**
CALORIES

29 g
Fat

36 g
Carbs

10 g
Protein

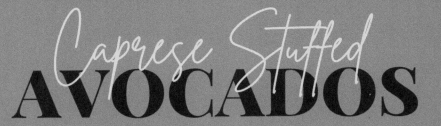

Caprese Stuffed AVOCADOS

INGREDIENTS

- 1 avocado
- ¼ cup cherry tomatoes
- ¼ cup mini mozzarella balls
- 1½ tbsp balsamic vinegar
- 1 tbsp olive oil

DIRECTIONS

1. Scoop out a little bit of an avocado to create a deeper pit.

2. Combine the cherry tomatoes and mozzarella balls in a bowl, then transfer them into the avocado.

3. Drizzle with balsamic vinegar and olive oil. Sprinkle with salt and pepper to taste.

Nutritional Value:

515 CALORIES

45 g
Fat

20 g
Carbs

8 g
Protein

5 min
Prep

25 min
Cook

2
Servings *

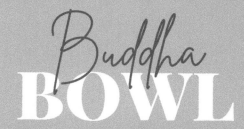

Buddha
BOWL

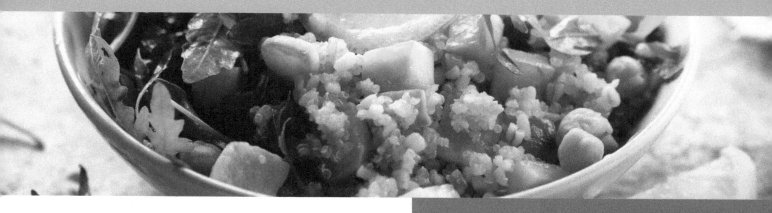

INGREDIENTS

- 4 cups spinach
- 1 cup quinoa
- 1 cup chickpeas
- 1 red bell pepper
- 1 cup cucumber
- 2 tbsp olive oil
- 2 tbsp lemon juice

Nutritional Value:

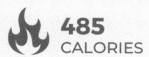 **485**
CALORIES

19 g
Fat

65 g
Carbs

16 g
Protein

DIRECTIONS

1. Prepare the quinoa by following the instructions provided on the packaging.

2. While the quinoa is cooking prepare all the vegetables and place them in a bowl.

3. Once everything is in the bowl, drizzle the lemon juice and olive oil on top. Sprinkle with salt and pepper to taste.

* Refrigerate one serving.

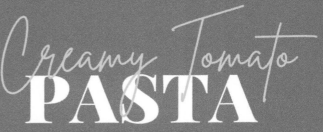

5 min
Prep

25 min
Cook

2
Servings *

Creamy Tomato PASTA

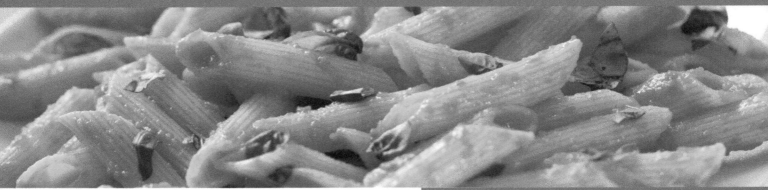

INGREDIENTS

- 7 oz brown rice pasta
- 2 red peppers
- 4 sun dried tomatoes
- 1 cup canned diced tomatoes
- ½ cup cashews
- 1 tbsp olive oil
- ¼ cup onions

DIRECTIONS

1. Soak the cashews in water for 2 hours. Prepare pasta according to instructions.

2. Heat pan with olive oil, onion, red pepper. Sauté 2-3 minute[s]

3. In a blender, combine tomatoes, cashews, sautéed vegetables. Blend until crean[y]

4. Add pasta to a bowl with sauce. Combine well, serve with fresh parsley on top.

* *Refrigerate one serving.*

Nutritional Value:

 **498**
CALORIES

22 g
Fat

63 g
Carbs

13 g
Protein

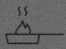 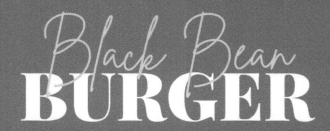

5 min
Prep

10 min
Cook

2 Servings *

Black Bean
BURGER

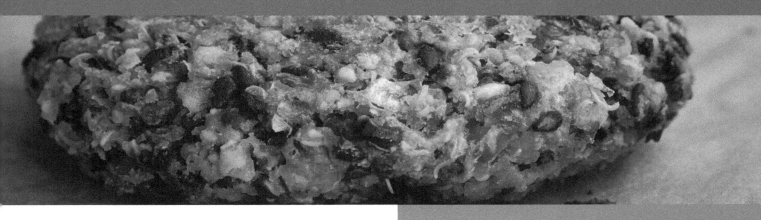

INGREDIENTS

- 1 ½ cups black beans
- ¼ cup gluten-free oats
- ¼ cup onion
- ¼ cup parsley
- 1 tsp chili powder
- 1 tsp coconut oil
- ½ tsp cumin
- 1 garlic clove

Nutritional Value:

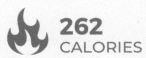 **262** CALORIES

2 g Fat

46 g Carbs

16 g Protein

DIRECTIONS

1. Drain black beans. Place all the ingredients and salt to taste in a food processor until the mixture becomes sticky.

2. Form 4 patties and cook on the stove top on medium heat with coconut oil.

3. Fry the patty for 3-5 minutes on each side and then you can add any of your favorite toppings to the burger patties.

* Refrigerate one serving.

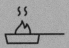

10 min
Prep

45 min
Cook

2
Servings *

Sweet Potato
CHICKPEA CURRY

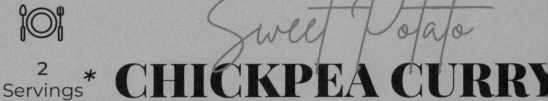

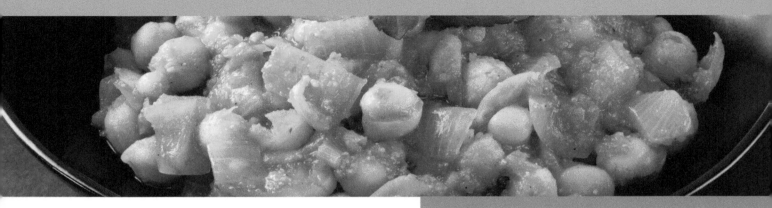

INGREDIENTS

- 1 sweet potato
- 1 can chickpeas
- 1 cup coconut milk
- ¼ cup onion
- 1 can tomato
- 1 tbsp olive oil
- 1 tbsp turmeric
- 1 tbsp cumin
- 1 tbsp ginger

DIRECTIONS

1. In a large pot heat olive oil, onions, spices, salt to taste. Cook until onions become translucent.

2. Add in the rest of the ingredients.

3. Bring the curry to a boil and then turn it down to a simmer for about 40 minutes or until the sweet potatoes are completely done.

* Refrigerate one serving.

Nutritional Value:

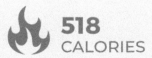 **518**
CALORIES

26 g
Fat

56 g
Carbs

13 g
Protein

5 min
Prep

 55 min
Cook

 2
Servings *

Stuffed
SWEET POTATO

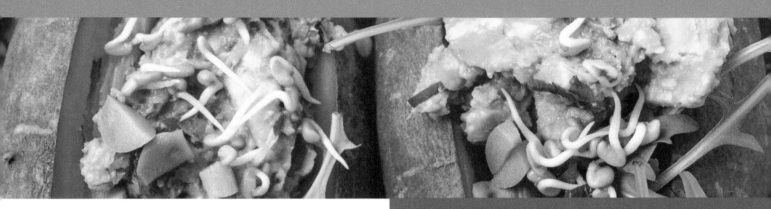

INGREDIENTS

- 2 sweet potatoes
- 1 cup black beans
- 1 cup corn
- 1 avocado
- 2 tomatoes
- ½ cup cilantro
- ¼ cup onion
- 2 tbsp lime juice

Nutritional Value:

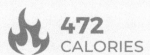 **472**
CALORIES

13 g
Fat

77 g
Carbs

16 g
Protein

DIRECTIONS

1. Preheat the oven to 425°F. Scrub the potatoes and pierce holes all around them with a fork. Bake in the oven for 45-50 minutes.

2. Combine the black beans and corn in one bowl. In a separate bowl, combine tomatoes, cilantro, onion, lime juice.

3. Stuff it with bean mixture, top it with sauce, avocado.

* *Refrigerate one serving.*

-35-

5 min
Prep

35 min
Cook

2
Servings

*

Lentil MEATBALLS

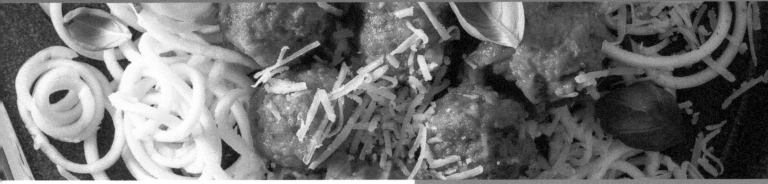

INGREDIENTS

- 3 large zucchinis
- 1 cup canned lentils
- ¼ cup quinoa
- ½ cup almond flour
- 1 tsp olive oil
- ¼ cup onion
- 2 garlic cloves
- 2 tbsp Italian seasoning
- 2 cups marinara sauce

DIRECTIONS

1. Prepare quinoa according to directions on the package.

2. Add everything except for the marinara sauce and zucchini in the food processor. Process until it is completely smooth. Roll out 10 small "meatballs".

3. Heat olive oil in pan, cook the meatballs for 5 minutes. Add sauce, cook for 5 minutes. Serve over spiralized zucchini

* Refrigerate one serving.

Nutritional Value:

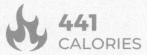 **441**
CALORIES

18 g
Fat

55 g
Carbs

20 g
Protein

5 min
Prep

15 min
Cook

2
Servings *

Kelp Noodle
STIR FRY

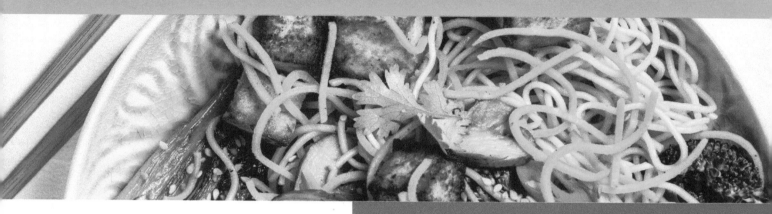

INGREDIENTS

- 10 oz tempeh
- 1 head broccoli
- 2 carrots
- ¼ cup onions
- 2 garlic cloves
- 1 tsp coconut oil
- 7 oz kelp noodles
- ¼ cup coconut aminos

Nutritional Value:

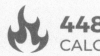 **448**
CALORIES

24 g
Fat

38 g
Carbs

35 g
Protein

DIRECTIONS

1. Heat pan and add coconut oil, onions and garlic. Once onions are translucent add the chopped broccoli, carrots. Cover and cook. Once the vegetables are cooked through add in the tempeh and cook for 3-5 minutes.

2. Add the coconut aminos, the kelp noodles, cover, and cook for an additional 2 minutes.

* *Refrigerate one serving.*

5 min Prep

25 min Cook

2 Servings *

PAD THAI
Tofu

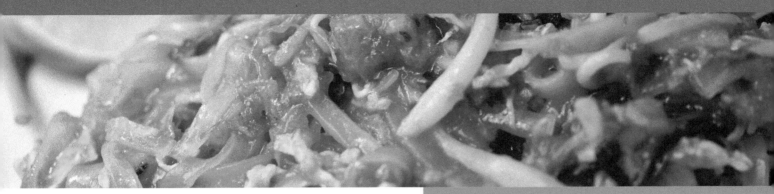

INGREDIENTS

- 7 oz tofu, cubed
- 3.5 oz brown rice noodles
- 1 cup bean sprouts
- 2 tbsp green onions
- ¼ cup coconut aminos
- 2 tbsp almond butter
- 1 tbsp coconut oil

DIRECTIONS

1. Prepare noodles according to directions on the package.

2. Place a pan on medium heat and add the coconut oil. Add in the tofu. Cook for 3 minutes add in sprouts. Mix coconut aminos, almond butter and toss it in pan, lower the heat. Cook for another 5 minutes.

3. Toss noodles in the pan, mix well. Top with green onions

* *Refrigerate one serving.*

Nutritional Value:

 **485** CALORIES

26 g	58 g	24 g
Fat	Carbs	Protein

-38-

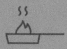 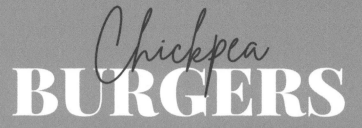

5 min
Prep

10 min
Cook

1
Serving

Chickpea
BURGERS

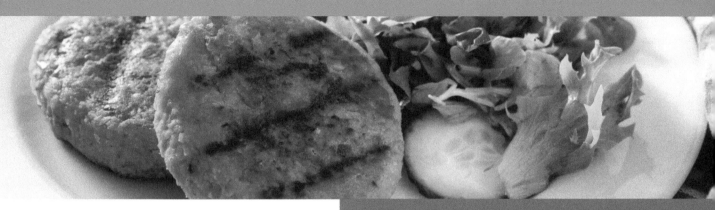

INGREDIENTS

- 6 oz (canned) chickpeas
- ¼ tbsp cumin
- 1 egg
- ¼ medium onion
- 1 tsp olive oil
- ½ cucumber
- ½ cup lettuce
- 1 tbsp breadcrumbs

Nutritional Value:

 **331**
CALORIES

9 g
Fat

37 g
Carbs

14 g
Protein

DIRECTIONS

1. In a food processor, blend the chickpeas, cumin, the egg and salt to taste. Put into a bowl and mix with breadcrumbs and the diced onions. Form 2 small burgers.

2. Heat the oil in a pan. Fry the burgers for 3-5 minutes each side. Serve with cucumber slices and lettuce.

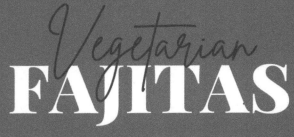

5 min
Prep

10 min
Cook

1
Serving

Vegetarian
FAJITAS

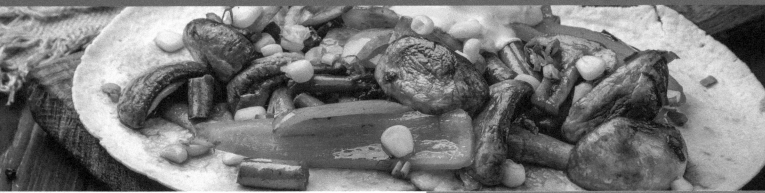

INGREDIENTS

- 1 tsp olive oil
- ¼ large onion
- ½ bell peppers
- ½ cup mushrooms
- Brown rice tortilla
- ¼ tsp paprika
- ¼ tsp onion powder
- ¼ cup black beans

Nutritional Value:

 **261**
CALORIES

7 g
Fat

33 g
Carbs

8 g
Protein

DIRECTIONS

1. Preheat pan. Add in oil, sliced onions and peppers. Saute for 4-5 minutes.

2. Add in sliced mushrooms, spices, salt to taste. Saute for 4-5 minutes longer. Add beans and stir to warm them through.

3. Serve on top of tortillas.

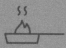

5 min
Prep

30 min
Cook

1
Serving

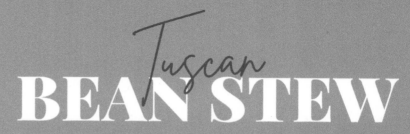

Tuscan
BEAN STEW

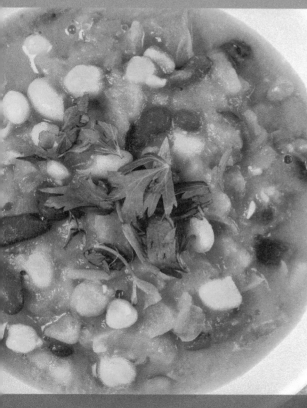

INGREDIENTS

- 1 tsp olive oil
- ¼ clove garlic
- 1 small carrot
- ½ stick celery
- ½ small leek, chopped
- 2 oz kale
- 1 cup vegetable broth
- 1 tsp tomato purée
- 6 oz (canned) borlotti beans

DIRECTIONS

1. Heat oil in a pan, add the garlic, leeks, carrot, celery and cook until softened. Add broth, tomato purée. Bring to a simmer, cook for 20 minutes. Add greens, beans and simmer for 5 more minutes.

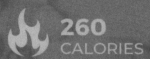

Nutritional Value:

260 CALORIES

6 g Fat

26 g Carbs

14 g Protein

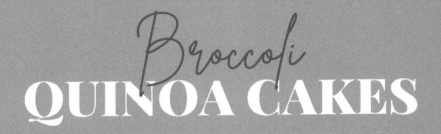

Broccoli
QUINOA CAKES

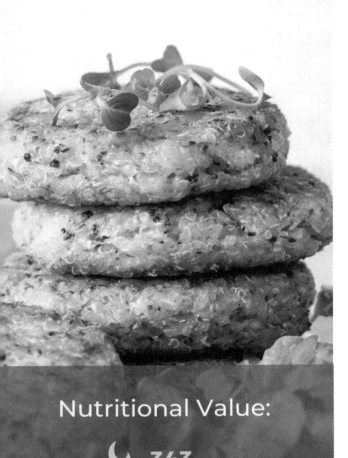

Nutritional Value:

343 CALORIES

17 g Fat   24 g Carbs   17 g Protein

INGREDIENTS

- ½ cup cooked quinoa
- 1 cup broccoli florets
- 1 green onion
- ¼ cup fresh herbs
- 1 egg
- ½ garlic clove
- ⅛ cup almond flour
- 1 tbsp grated cheese
- 1 tsp olive oil
- ¼ cup lettuce
- ¼ cup shredded red cabbage

DIRECTIONS

1. Steam the broccoli until tender. Place broccoli, herbs, cooked quinoa, egg, salt to taste, garlic, green onion and cheese into a food processor and pulse repeatedly until finely ground. Pulse in the almond flour, mixing in well. Form 2 patties.

2. Heat the oil in a pan. Fry the patties for 5 minutes each side. Serve with lettuce, shredded red cabbage.

Hummus & CUCUMBERS

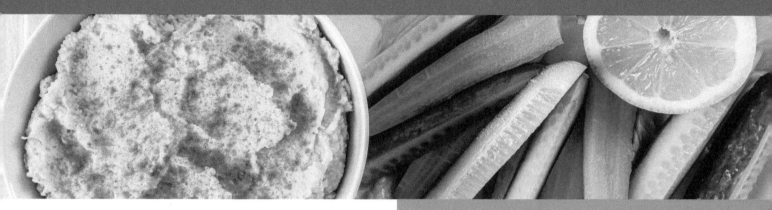

INGREDIENTS

- 1 can chickpeas
- ¼ cup tahini
- 2 tbsp olive oil
- 2 tbsp lemon juice
- 1 tsp cumin
- 1 english cucumber
- 1 garlic clove

Nutritional Value:

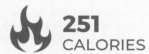 **251** CALORIES

16 g
Fat

22 g
Carbs

8 g
Protein

DIRECTIONS

1. Drain the chickpeas and rinse them well.

2. Place all the ingredients and salt to taste in a food processor and process until it forms a smooth and creamy texture.

3. Store the hummus into an air-tight container or portion it out immediately into 4 servings.

5 min
Prep

 1
Serving

Carrots &
ALMOND BUTTER

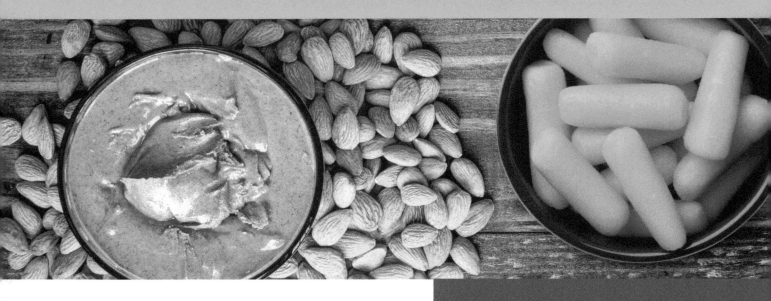

INGREDIENTS

- 2 carrots
- 1 tbsp almond butter

Nutritional Value:

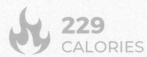 **229**
CALORIES

19 g
Fat

13 g
Carbs

5 g
Protein

DIRECTIONS

1. Slice the carrots into sticks and use the almond butter as a dip.

-44-

5 min
Prep

45 min
Cook

4
Servings

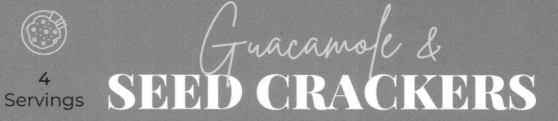

Guacamole &
SEED CRACKERS

INGREDIENTS

- ¼ cup chia seeds
- ¼ cup sesame seeds
- ¼ cup sunflower seeds
- ½ tbsp herb mix seasoning
- ½ mashed avocado
- Juice of ½ lime

DIRECTIONS

1. Combine all the seeds with 1 cup water and seasonings. Let the mixture sit for 5 minutes

2. Preheat the oven to 325°F. Spread the seed mixture evenly until flat. Bake for 30 minutes then remove from the oven, cut them into squares, flip them and bake for another 15 minutes.

3. Combine mashed avocado and lime juice, salt to taste and mash.

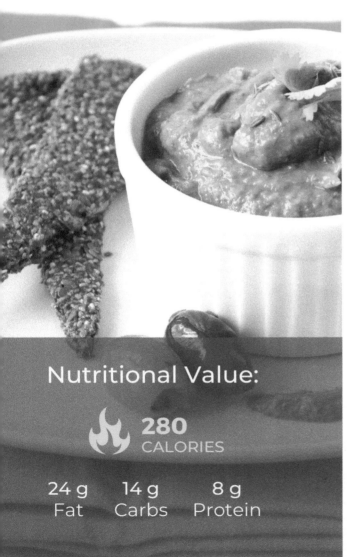

Nutritional Value:

280 CALORIES

24 g Fat

14 g Carbs

8 g Protein

Cacao
COCONUT BALLS

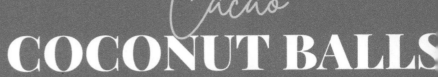

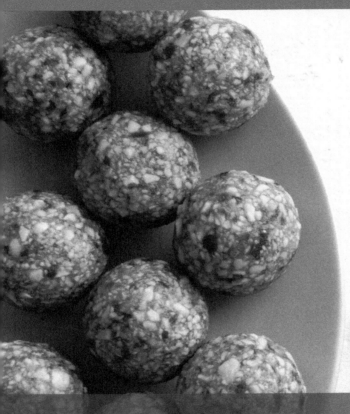

INGREDIENTS

- 1 cup almonds
- ½ cup shredded coconut
- 8 medjool dates
- 2 tbsp raw cacao powder

DIRECTIONS

1. Remove the pit from the dates. Combine all the ingredients in a food processor and mix until it forms a doughy mixture.

2. Form 10 balls with the mixture and then store them in the fridge to preserve freshness.

Nutritional Value:
For 2 balls

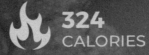 **324**
CALORIES

18 g
Fat

36 g
Carbs

6 g
Protein

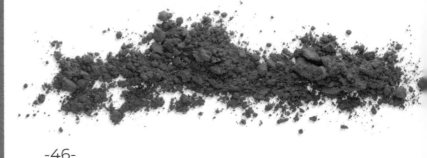

5 min
Prep

5 min
Cook

5
Servings

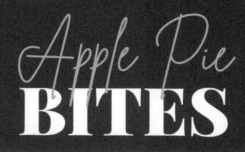

Apple Pie
BITES

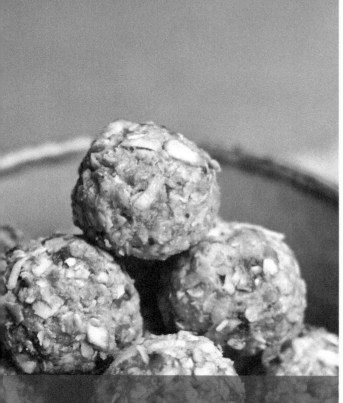

INGREDIENTS

- 8 medjool dates
- 1 cup dried apples
- 1 cup walnuts
- 1 tsp ground cinnamon

DIRECTIONS

1. Remove the pit from the dates. Combine all the ingredients in a food processor and mix until it forms a doughy mixture.

2. Form 10 balls with the mixture and then store them in the fridge to preserve freshness.

Nutritional Value:
For 2 balls

 314
CALORIES

16 g
Fat

44 g
Carbs

5 g
Protein

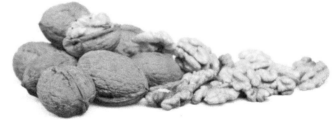

Superfood COOKIES

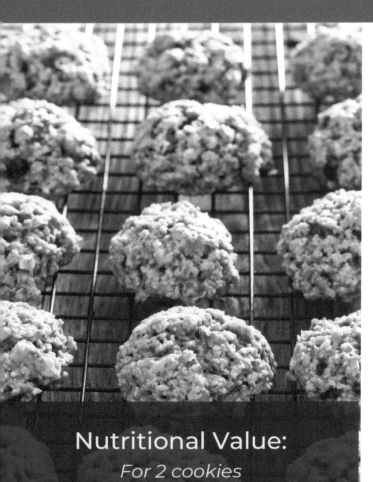

Nutritional Value:

For 2 cookies

468 CALORIES

24 g	56 g	10 g
Fat	Carbs	Protein

INGREDIENTS

- 1 ½ cup gluten-free rolled oats
- ¼ cup dried cranberries
- ¼ cup pumpkin seeds
- 1 banana
- 2 tbsp ground flax seeds
- 2 tbsp chia seeds
- ¼ cup maple syrup
- ¼ cup coconut oil

DIRECTIONS

1. Combine all the dry ingredients in a medium bowl. In a separate bowl, mash the banana, then add the melted coconut oil and maple syrup.

2. Preheat the oven to 325°F. Combine the dry and wet ingredients and form 8 cookies. Bake the cookies for 18 minutes

Easy
TRAIL MIX

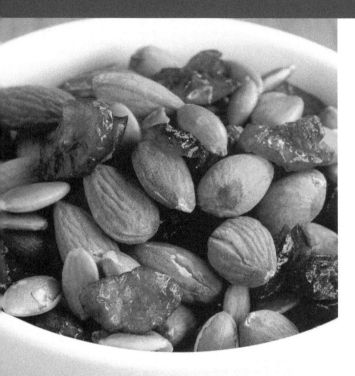

INGREDIENTS

- ¼ cup dried cranberries
- ¼ cup almonds
- ¼ cup pumpkin seeds
- ½ cup coconut chips

DIRECTIONS

1. Place all the ingredients in an air-tight jar and store somewhere cool or immediately divide the trail mix into 3 portions.

Nutritional Value:

 **256**
CALORIES

20 g
Fat

9 g
Carbs

10 g
Protein

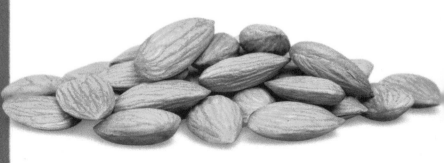

5 min
Prep

2 hours
Cook

1
Serving

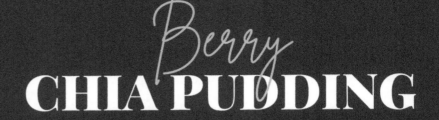

Berry
CHIA PUDDING

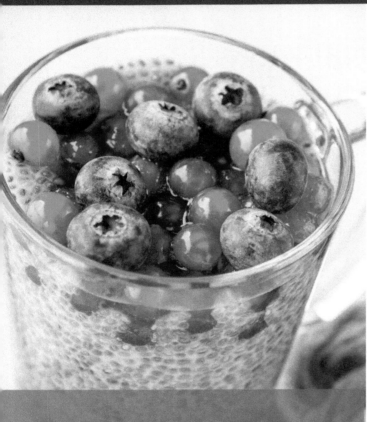

INGREDIENTS

- 2 tbsp chia seeds
- ½ cup almond milk
- 1 tsp maple syrup
- 1 cup mixed berries

DIRECTIONS

1. Place the chia seeds, almond milk, and maple syrup in an air-tight jar and mix well.

2. Place in the fridge to set for at least 2 hours or overnight. Serve with fresh berries.

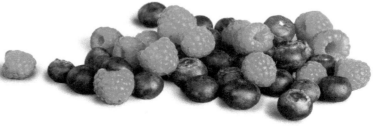

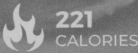

Nutritional Value:

221
CALORIES

11 g
Fat

29 g
Carbs

6 g
Protein

Ingram Content Group UK Ltd.
Milton Keynes UK
UKHW050935040523
421173UK00003B/31

9 798987 352090